MW00875049

What Do You See?

Painting the Picture in Hospice Documentation for Eligibility

Michelle Crowell 2016

Michelle Crowell has been in the nursing field for 23 years with the last 15 years in hospice. Held CHPN certification from 2006-2010. Has served in many leadership positions and currently serves as a state administrator over 17 hospices. She has a passion for hospice patients and for hospice nurses and her desire is each nurse has the proper resources necessary to adequately prove hospice eligibility.

As a new nurse in hospice, oftentimes it is difficult to understand the language needed to properly document hospice eligibility. My goal is writing this companion book was to give examples of what is needed for disease documentation. It is truly about painting the picture. I will list items that need to be included in your documentation along with examples of generalized documentation versus specific and appropriate documentation.

The following categories of functional status, nutritional status, pain and mental status are very important to document on each individual no matter disease process and will play a huge part in proving eligibility. Also it is very important to document co-morbidities as they correlate most of the time directly with the primary diagnosis and prognosis of the patient.

Functional Status:

- How do they move around? Do they ambulate? Are they bedbound?

- Do they require an assistive device? Do they require assistance from others?

- Do they have contractures?

- How is their gait? Have they had any falls?

- Have they had changes in their need for assistance with ADLS?

- What is their PPS, FAST or KPS score?

In this section it is important to document the true level of their functional status. The PPS/KPS scores are important to use to gauge where a person is at. Also let's say the person may be sitting up in a chair but do we show the level that it took for them to be in that position. Did it require 3 persons to sit them in that chair? Are they propped up on each side with pillows? Do you get the picture now?

They are in the chair but not independently?

Nutritional Status:

- Appetite level? Do not put poor, fair or good. This is generalized and does not truly show the level of a patient's intake. Are they eating 25% of two meals daily? Do they drop portions of their food due to hands shaking? Are they pocketing the food in the side of their mouth?

- Are they only in taking liquids? Ice chips only? Have they completely stopped eating?

- Do they require to be fed? Does their food need pureed or specialized?

- Are they being fed by Peg/Gtube? If so what is the type of feeding, continuous or intermittent? Do they have residual? Are they aspirating? Are they bloated? How does the site of the tube look?

- Is there any nausea/vomiting, diarrhea/constipation? Describe each one. What medications are you giving for intervention? Reaction, side effects, understanding of medication usage.

- Reasons for possible poor appetite-mouth sores/ulcers, loose or ill-fitting dentures.

- Bowel sounds- present/not present-hypo/hyperactive or normal.

- Difficulty swallowing? Reasons for? Any interventions?

- Supplements? Type? Amount? Frequency?

- Abdominal ascites/distention? What is girth measurement?

- Is there weight loss? Arm or thigh circumference loss?

- If unable to weigh have they loss size in clothing, size in diaper wear

- Is their face sunken or gaunt in appearance?

- What interventions are you doing for any of these items above?

Nutrition is very important to show an overall decline in the condition of the patient. Be very specific in the documentation of this category. There is a huge difference in saying the patient has a poor appetite versus saying the patient is only able to consume 15% at best of two meals in which they often drop part of their food on the floor due to unsteady hand. Or saying the patient is losing weight vs the patient has went from wearing a size large in clothing to a medium and down from a large depend to a medium. Can you picture the patient is not getting the proper nutrition needed?

Pain:

- Most nursing assessments deal with pain assessment as this has become a big component in CMS review of quality management of this symptom.

- Monitor pain each visit and as needed.

- Monitor if pain, what is the pain level? Location, type, what increases the pain? What relieves the pain?

- What interventions are you doing? Are they successful?

- What medications are you using? Does the patient/patient care giver understand the medication, use of, side effects, how to properly administer medication?

- Are you documenting non medication interventions such as repositioning of patient, sounds and imagery, diversion and other interventions?

Skin/Wounds:

- How does the skin look in appearance? Pale, discolored, mottled, jaundiced?

- Are they any lesions? Skin tears? Bruising?

- Skin temperature?

- Does the patient have an IV access? How does the site look? Describe site, appearance, type of access, medication being infused, and family understanding of the site and signs and symptoms to report of any abnormalities.

- Are there any wound? Describe type of wound, location, appearance, odor, drainage, tunneling or not, wound care instructions and understanding by caregiver on wound care.

- Have you measured the wounds? Noted improvement or decline?

- Is the skin weeping? Excessive sweating? Odor?

- Is there any edema? Describe location. Is it pitting? Dependent?

Urinary & Bowels

- Is patient incontinent? Bladder? Bowels?

- Does patient have a Foley? Size? Date of last catheter change?
  How does urine look?

- Date of last bowel movement? Any abnormalities?

- Any constipation, diarrhea, impaction? Any urine retention? Dysuria? Hematuria? Decrease in urine output?

Neurological:

- Assess patient level of consciousness. Are they oriented?

- Confusion? Agitation? Depression/anxiety? Combative?

- Assess speech? Do they have difficulty talking? Aphasic? Are their words garbled, inappropriate? Are they non-responsive?

- How does the patient sleep?

- Any interventions for any of the items above?

All of the items that we have discussed so far are all necessary to discuss for the overall status of a patient. The items we will look at now will be geared toward patient disease specific documentation. I will briefly cover the top 3 non cancer diagnosis used in hospice.

Cardiac disease:

With any type of end stage heart disease, CHF, Atrial fibrillation or any other disease processes that may fall under this category it is very important to document specific to the disease process.

- Heart rate? Irregular? Murmur? Faint? Strong?

- Was pulse rate apical, carotid, radial, or pedal?

- Edema in face, eyes, extremities? Type? Pitting? Non pitting?

- Abdominal girth? Many heart patients will hold fluid in abdomen.

- Chest pain? Location? Type? Length it last? What makes it better? Worse? Taking any Nitroglycerin? How often?

- Shortness of breath? With what type of exertion? At rest? What makes better? What makes worse? O2? Amount of O2?

- Clubbing? Jugular vein distention? Capillary refill?

- Sleep functions? Physical Endurance?

- Medications and Interventions taken?

- NYHA scale-level 4 is needed to be hospice appropriate.

Respiratory disease:

- Lung sounds- Rhonchi? Rales? Wheezes? Diminished? Which lung fields?

- Shortness of breath? Exertion? At rest? Can they talk without getting short of breath?

- Respiratory rate and pattern? Cheyne Stokes? Labored? Apnea?

- Coughing? Productive/nonproductive?

- O2? Rate? Continuous or Prn?

- Barrel chest? Using accessory muscles to breathe?

- Inhalers? Respiratory nebulizer treatments? Kinds, amounts, frequencies?

Alzheimer's disease:

This disease process is truly focused on functional status, nutritional status and level of comprehension. The FAST score must be 7. Documentation should show that the patient is unable to carry on a sensible conversation of 6 words or more. They may speak more words but they must be garbled, word salad, incomprehensible or do not make sense to the questions being asked.

Examples of proper documentation for hospice eligibility:

In order to prove eligibility to CMS for hospice coverage, each form of documentation must state their case and must stand alone. Comprehensive assessments completed on admission by the RN, as well as recertification visits, physician's narratives for certification process and each individual disciplines' notes must show that the patient meets and continues to meet eligibility. It is all about giving you credit for what you have assessed and implemented. We must learn to document in specific terms so that we will speak in the same manner. Oftentimes the physician will document based on the language we use. If we use generalities, then that is the type of documentation that will be completed. I will list several forms of appropriate versus inappropriate documentation. My hope is that you will be able to see how to gear your level of thinking toward painting the picture of true decline in your patients.

#1 Generalized Documentation- Not appropriate: Patient gets short of breath while walking. Uses oxygen. Coughs at times.

#1 Detailed/Specific Documentation- appropriate: Patient has disabling dyspnea after only ambulating 10 feet with a walker before having to sit down and requires a 10-minute recovery time before resuming ambulating the last 10 feet to the living room. Patient has O2 @ 2L/min BNC continuously. Using Albuterol nebulizer treatments four times a day to help increase open airways. Has productive cough of clear thick sputum.

#2 Generalized Documentation- Not appropriate: Patient's appetite has decreased. Not eating well. Looks to have lost weight but unable to weigh.

#2 Detailed/Specific Documentation- appropriate: Patient has gone from eating 50% of 3 meals daily to only eating at best 25% of 2 meals and often only takes 2-3 bites at each meal setting. Requires to be fed by caregiver and often spits food out or has difficulty swallowing. Intakes liquids easier if thickened. Supplemented with Ensure twice daily of 4oz. Patient is unable to weigh but has lost 0.5cm in mid arm circumference of the right upper arm and has lost 1cm of right thigh mid circumference. Patient has also gone down one size in clothing and diaper size. Eyes have sunken look to them. Skin turgor is >3 seconds

#3 Generalized Documentation- Not appropriate: Patient is actively dying and is not doing well. Has had a change in body processes.

Detailed/Specific Documentation- appropriate: Patient has entered the active dying process. Patient is non responsive to verbal or tactile stimuli but will moan and groan to painful stimuli. Patient has not eaten in 3 days

and has only taken in a few ice chips of liquid during that time. Urinary output has decreased. Patient has temperature of 101.6F and skin is beginning to mottle in the bend of the knee and across the lower back area.

Can you see? It is all about painting the picture. If I close my eyes and read your documentation can I visualize the patient and the progression of the disease process that their body is experiencing? Can I prove they meet hospice criteria? Documentation is the key to not only proving eligibility but to ensuring proper care and interventions are being implemented. Although I could list hundreds of documented wrong vs right, I hope that this simple booklet will get you thinking about your documentation.

What does your canvas look like? What do you see?